Anna Miller

Healing Seeds

Transforming Health with Psyllium

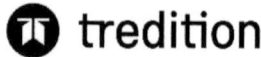 tredition

© 2024, Anna Miller (2nd Edition)

Druck und Distribution im Auftrag des Autors:
tredition GmbH, Heinz-Beusen-Stieg 5, 22926 Ahrensburg, Deutschland

Das Werk, einschließlich seiner Teile, ist urheberrechtlich geschützt. Für die Inhalte ist die Autorin verantwortlich. Jede Verwertung ist ohne ihre Zustimmung unzulässig. Die Publikation und Verbreitung erfolgen im Auftrag der Autorin, zu erreichen unter: tredition GmbH, Abteilung "Impressumservice", Heinz-Beusen-Stieg 5, 22926 Ahrensburg, Deutschland

Contents

PSYLLIUM: THE PATH TO HEALTH AND HAPPINESS - A TRUE STORY OF TRANSFORMATION 9

Introduction 9

The dark times 12

The discovery of psyllium 14

The beginning of change 16

The positive effects on digestion 19

A new chapter of well-being 21

The return to normality 23

The passion for psyllium 25

The dissemination of knowledge 27

A sustainable change 30

Conclusion 33

PSYLLIUM: THE NATURAL SOURCE FOR HEALTH AND WELL-BEING 38

Introduction 38

Chapter 1: The health benefits of psyllium 46

Chapter 2: Weight management with psyllium 50

Chapter 3: Cardiovascular Health and Psyllium 54

Chapter 4: Diabetes management with psyllium 60

Chapter 5: Psyllium for healthy intestinal flora 64

Chapter 6: Detoxification and cleansing of the body with psyllium 68

Chapter 7: Skin health and psyllium 72

Chapter 8: Psyllium in children's nutrition 75

Chapter 9: Tips for using psyllium in the kitchen 79

Conclusion 84

PSYLLIUM CUISINE: HEALTHY RECIPES FOR EVERY MEAL 88

Introduction 88

Chapter 1: Breakfast ideas 92

Chapter 2: Appetizers and snacks 96

Chapter 3: Soups and salads 101

Chapter 4: Main dishes - Vegetarian and Vegan 106

Chapter 5: Main dishes - meat and fish 111

Chapter 6: Side dishes and side salads 116

Chapter 7: Snacks 121

Chapter 8: Recipes for toddlers 125

Chapter 9: Sweet treats and desserts 129

Chapter 10: Drinks with psyllium 135

Chapter 11: Psyllium for external use 139

Chapter 12: Recipes for pets 143

Psyllium: The Path to Health and Happiness - A True Story of Transformation

Introduction

Dear Readers,

My story is one of overcoming health issues, looking for healing, and ultimately discovering the transformative power of psyllium. I would like to make it known to you now. This report was written by me, Anna Muller, and my name is Anna Muller. My life, which was characterized by the shadows of an invisible disease, is disclosed in a manner that is both honest and personal.

I have been plagued by excruciating gastrointestinal complaints that have impacted my day-to-day life ever since I was a child. Constipation, diarrhea, bloating, and abdominal pain were constant companions for me despite my best efforts. When it comes to never knowing when or how severe these symptoms will be, I cannot stress enough how frustrating and limiting it is to be in this situation.

I experienced feelings of helplessness on occasion. In addition to having a physical impact on me, the anxiety and insecurity that accompanied it also had an emotional impact. As I became more reclusive and avoided engaging in social activities in order to avoid embarrassing situations, I found that the joy that come from the simple things in life began to fade.

In an effort to find a treatment, I set out on a very difficult journey. On the other hand, despite numerous trips to the physician and medical examinations, conclusive answers were not obtained. Irritable bowel syndrome was diagnosed, which didn't stop the questions from coming. I felt as though I was stuck in a never-ending cycle, and conventional treatments did not provide any relief that would last.

Now, however, I am aware of psyllium. A natural remedy that was praised by a minority of individuals. Confession: I had some reservations. Were I not already subjected to a great deal of dissatisfaction? So I made the decision to give it a shot. As a result, I decided to take control of my own health and not make any further concessions.

My experience with psyllium started off with this. My experiences far surpassed any and all expectations I had. My symptoms gradually started to improve day by day. I felt lighter and more energized, and my digestion was regulated. The pain also subsided.

However, the most significant of all was that I was able to regain my enthusiasm for life. The feeling of being able to actively participate in life once more without being overshadowed by the shadows of my illness is so liberating that I am unable to adequately describe it to you. Psyllium was instrumental in assisting me in regaining my health and putting me on the path to living a life that is rich in joy and fulfillment.

Through this report, I hope to encourage you, show you that there is always hope, and share with you the journey that I have been on. Let's open the door to health and happiness by discovering together the transformative power of psyllium, which it possesses.

The dark times

There are times when the past appears to be a gloomy shadow that exerts a burden on us, causing our lives to descend into an endless darkness. These difficult times started for me many years ago, when my health problems reached the point where they became an ever-present burden.

To this day, I can still pinpoint the exact moment when I experienced the first symptoms of irritable bowel syndrome, which completely turned my life upside down. The abdominal pain, which at first glance appeared to be benign, eventually turned into a daily struggle that gradually diminished my enthusiasm for life. I had the impression that my body was conspiring against me, as if it wanted to tell me over and over again, "You can't just live a normal life like this."

The effect that it had on my life was heartbreaking. As I moved forward, I was constantly plagued by the worry that the next episode of diarrhea or constipation would come as a complete surprise to me. These social activities, which I used to take great pleasure in, have turned into a minefield of humiliation and insecurity for me. Maintaining an appearance of strength on the outside while I was breaking down on the inside was a challenge that I faced on a consistent basis.

It was difficult to cope with the overwhelming feelings of frustration and hopelessness that accompanied my search for relief and healing. In the hope that I would finally be able to find answers, I allowed myself to be dragged from one doctor to another and from one examination to another. However, the majority of the findings were consistently the same: there were no organic causes and no obvious solutions.

My search for information on the Internet lasted for countless hours, and I looked for other people who had experienced something comparable to what I had. I did not want to be by myself; I wanted to be aware that I was not the only person who was afflicted with this disease that was not visible to the naked eye. However, at the same time, the never-ending posts on the forum and the testimonials made me feel even more hopeless. As far as I could tell, there was no genuine possibility of recovery.

The dark times were characterized by feelings of anxiety and self-doubt. Whether or not I would ever be able to lead a normal life, whether or not I would ever be liberated from the chains of this suffering, I pondered the possibility. However, despite the fact that I was in the midst of this darkness, there was a glimmer of hope that kept me going. The conviction that there must be a solution somewhere in the world, even if I had not yet discovered it, was the source of this belief.

As we move forward into the subsequent chapters, I would like to take you on a journey with me through the difficult times and into the bright light of transformation. It is a tale of perseverance, adversity, and ultimately, the process of healing. Discovering the path that brought me to psyllium and opened a new chapter of happiness is something that we should do together.

The discovery of psyllium

On a day that seemed like any other, I happened upon something that would forever alter the course of my life. When I was trying to find information about irritable bowel syndrome (IBS), I remember researching it on the internet. An article that was relatively brief and unassuming discussed the potential advantages of psyllium for the treatment of gastrointestinal distress. My curiosity was piqued, but I also had some reservations about it.

Psyllium? Was it possible that something so uncomplicated and natural could actually be the answer to my years of suffering? Already, I had tried a great number of purported treatments, only to be let down by the results. Before the symptoms returned, the majority of them had only provided me with temporary relief.

Even though I had some reservations, I made the decision to learn more about psyllium. Reading studies, looking through testimonials, and even having conversations with individuals who had positive experiences with this natural remedy were all things that I did. Little by little, a glimmer of optimism started to light up inside of me.

Putting aside my long-standing reservations about natural remedies was not an easy task for me to accomplish. I was no longer able to have faith in conventional medicine, and I often felt as though it had abandoned me. Nevertheless, I came to the realization that it was time to be open to new opportunities. The idea that there was nothing to lose by giving psyllium a shot was something that I had to persuade myself against.

To this day, I can vividly recall the day that I purchased my very first packet of psyllium. At the time, it seemed like a minor act of departure, a step in a direction that was not known. At the same time that I was hopeful and nervous, I was wondering if I had finally discovered something that could alleviate the discomfort that I was experiencing.

My first encounter with psyllium seeds will be described in the following paragraphs, along with the profound effect that these seeds had on my life and how they influenced my life in general. There is a transformation that takes place in this story, which demonstrates that sometimes the most straightforward solutions can be the most effective. Let's go on an adventure together and discover the path that brought me to a fresh understanding of my health and, ultimately, brought me back to living a life that is rich and full of joy.

The beginning of change

My choice to experiment with psyllium was not only one of the most challenging but also one of the most significant choices I have ever made in my life. After dealing with the symptoms of irritable bowel syndrome for such a long period of time, I was willing to try anything in order to find relief.

Still to this day, I can vividly recall standing in front of my very first dose of psyllium. The small amount of powder that I had in my palm had such a significant feeling. The object was a representation of optimism and fresh starts. With a resolute determination, I took the psyllium seeds and started my journey toward alleviation of the symptoms I was experiencing in my gastrointestinal tract.

I had a hard time believing what I was going through in the first few days and weeks after I started taking the psyllium in question. This natural source of fiber elicited a response from my body, and I had the sensation that my digestive system was being gently regulated. As time went on, the persistent abdominal pain became less severe, and the irregular bowel movements started to return to their normal pattern.

On the other hand, the psyllium itself was not the only factor that contributed to the change. It dawned on me that in order to achieve the best possible outcomes, I needed to make some changes to my diet. I started paying closer attention to the foods that I ate and discovered that certain foods were compounding the symptoms that I was experiencing. At a slow but steady pace, I constructed a diet that prioritized my well-being and the maintenance of a healthy digestive system.

There were times when it was difficult to make these adjustments. It required letting go of routine eating patterns as well as foods that were personal favorites. On the other hand, I was aware that it was necessary for both my physical and mental well-being. Over the course of time, I became adept at discovering new delectable dishes that were able to satiate both my taste buds and my stomach.

The changes that I experienced as a result of taking the psyllium and making necessary adjustments to my diet were not only noticeable on a physical level, but also on an emotional level. No longer did I experience a sense of helplessness and submission to my illness. Rather than that, I experienced a growing sense of strength and confidence that I could positively influence my own health on my own.

In the following paragraphs, I will share with you some of the additional experience I have gained along this path of transformation. This is a journey that is full of opportunities for discovery, triumphant moments, and challenges. In this article, we will discuss how psyllium and a conscious diet have had a long-lasting impact on my life and how they have helped me gradually become a version of myself that is liberated from the constraints of irritable bowel syndrome (IBS).

The positive effects on digestion

After I began incorporating psyllium into my daily routine, I gradually became aware of a significant improvement in the way that my digestion was functioning. The vexing digestive issues that had been plaguing me for years started to gradually disappear once I started to feel better.

The alleviation of the pain in my stomach was one of the first positive changes that I observed. When I was younger, I had the sensation that I was constantly carrying a heavy stone in my stomach, which dragged me down and deprived me of all of my energy. On the other hand, as time went on, the pain became somewhat less severe and occurred less frequently. I was finally able to concentrate on other things without being constantly distracted by my irritable digestive system. I was able to once again focus on other things.

I also noticed that my digestion became more consistent and reliable in general. When I was younger, I frequently experienced constipation, which was not only a physically unpleasant condition but also had a significant impact on both my mood and my overall well-being. Psyllium seeds, on the other hand, assisted in the natural emptying of my bowels, and I discovered a new equilibrium in my digestive system while using them.

The sense of relief and happiness that I experienced as a result of these enhancements is difficult to put into words. At long last, I was able to take pleasure in my life without having to constantly worry about my stomach and digestion. I experienced a sense of lightness, increased energy, and freedom to pursue my goals and dreams.

I was not only relieved from the physical pain, but I was also able to take action to improve the health of my intestinal tract, which was another factor that contributed to my happiness. I was able to regain control of my own body and was aware that I had discovered a potent instrument to enhance my overall health and wellness through the use of psyllium.

I will give you more information about the positive effects that this has had on my health and overall well-being in the following sections. Together, let's investigate how psyllium not only altered my physical appearance but also my emotional state, thereby enabling me to lead a life that is rich in vitality and happiness.

A new chapter of well-being

As each week went by, I experienced a sense of improved health and increased vitality. It would be impossible to ignore the significant positive effects that the psyllium has had on my body. I was able to sustainably improve my well-being, and I started to take pleasure in every moment of my life.

The increase in my energy was one of the most remarkable changes that took place. I used to frequently experience feelings of exhaustion and fatigue, even after a full night's sleep. However, by taking the psyllium, I was able to experience a newfound vitality that enabled me to begin each day with a sense of ease and enthusiasm. My ability to concentrate improved, I became more productive, and I experienced a sense of readiness to face the challenges that are inherent in everyday life.

In addition, this enhanced vitality manifested itself in my day-to-day activities. At long last, I was able to resume engaging in activities that I had neglected for a considerable amount of time. I was able to actively participate in my life, whether it was through a stroll through the park, a strenuous workout at the gym, or even just playing with my children. I possessed the strength and confidence to pursue these activities. The routine activities of my life turned into an exciting journey that I conquered with a sense of joy and enthusiasm.

On the other hand, not only did my physical life change, but so did my emotional life. I experienced a significant improvement in my emotional well-being as a result of the alleviation of long-standing complaints and the improvement in my physical health. I was finally able to laugh without any inhibitions, and I felt happier and more balanced as a result.

It is impossible to deny the influence that psyllium had on my life. My day-to-day life was liberated from a burden, and I was able to concentrate on fully appreciating the beautiful moments that were occurring. I discovered a new source of inner strength, which inspired me to pursue my dreams and accomplish my objectives, and my self-confidence increased as a result.

In the following paragraphs, I would like to provide you with additional information regarding the improvement in both my health and the quality of my life. I would like to discuss with you how psyllium has improved the quality of my life and provided me with the opportunity to fully realize the potential that lies within my existence.

The return to normality

The time had finally come; I had triumphed over my health issues, which had been a source of difficulty and impairment for many years. My discomfort was alleviated and I was able to return to my normal routine with the assistance of the psyllium.

Regaining the ability to lead a life that was completely normal, full of joy, and full of activity was an amazing sensation. My health was no longer a source of constant worry and restrictions; those days were finally over. At long last, I was able to take pleasure in each day without being hindered by either pain or discomfort.

The triumph over my health impairments allowed me to access previously unavailable opportunities and doors. It was possible for me to travel once more, to learn about new places, and to experience adventures that I had not previously considered to be possible. My interests and hobbies eventually became an essential component of my life, and I gained a more profound comprehension of the significance of maintaining a healthy and well-being lifestyle.

On the other hand, something had changed not only superficially but also internally. There had been a significant improvement in my emotional environment. I had been experiencing a sense of self-assurance and inner peace, which had replaced the worry and anxiety that had been weighing me down. Being able to see life through fresh eyes, I was able to comprehend how precious and valuable each and every moment was.

A turning point in my life occurred when I was able to return to normalcy. I came to the realization that I had the ability to influence both my physical well-being and my emotional state. For me, the psyllium had become a symbol of transformation, serving as a constant reminder of how far I had come and how powerful I had become with each passing day.

Within the following paragraphs, I intend to provide you with additional information regarding my journey and the manner in which I have incorporated psyllium into my life in order to enhance both my health and life quality. Let's investigate together how I have brought about a new normal in my life, as well as how you, too, can discover your own way to improved health and happiness.

The passion for psyllium

Having personally experienced the beneficial effects that psyllium seeds have had on my own health, I have become an ardent supporter of these seeds, which are relatively small but possess a great deal of power. My life has been transformed by them, and I am now a happier and healthier person as a result. Currently, I am interested in sharing my experience with others in order to assist them in reaping the benefits of psyllium seeds as well.

My enthusiasm for psyllium is difficult to put into words because of its effectiveness. This natural source of health has provided me with a new lease on life and has rid me of the ailments that I have been suffering from for a very long time. One of my greatest passions is assisting other people in experiencing their own personal transformation.

It is from the depths of my heart that I am inspired to tell you about my previous experiences. When I think back to that time, I do remember feeling exactly the same way: hopeless, frustrated, and looking for a solution. My health was restored through the use of psyllium, and I am confident that it is possible for other people to experience the same positive effects as I did.

It is my hope that I can inspire individuals to embark on their own journey and discover the opportunities that nature has to offer. The power of psyllium lies in the fact that it naturally stimulates the body's capacity for healing and provides support to the body. It is a method that is not only gentle and sustainable, but also lacks any adverse effects.

It is my hope that by sharing my story, other people will be motivated to experiment with new methods and investigate alternative methods. The number of people who are struggling with health problems is extremely high, and it is possible that they have not yet discovered the solution that they are looking for. My goal is to inspire them and demonstrate to them that there is still hope.

One of my deepest aspirations is to assist other people in starting their own journey toward health and happiness. Through the dissemination of my expertise and experience, I hope to make a constructive contribution and inspire others to take charge of their lives and realize their full potential.

The following sections will be dedicated to a more in-depth examination of the advantages and opportunities presented by psyllium. It is time for us to continue this journey together and explore the world of natural remedies in order to live a life that is both full and healthy.

The dissemination of knowledge

In my capacity as an ambassador for psyllium and healthy eating, I believe it is my duty to disseminate information about this wonderful plant and the benefits it offers. Now that I have personal experience with the profound impact that psyllium has had on my life, I am motivated to encourage other individuals to embark on their own personal health journeys.

When it comes to achieving happiness and realizing our full potential in life, it is incredible how much attention we sometimes need to pay to our health problems. The use of natural remedies such as psyllium, in addition to maintaining a healthy diet, has proven to be extremely beneficial, as I have discovered through my own personal experience.

My concern for the dissemination of this information has evolved into a matter of the heart. My experience has shown me that the lives of other people have been transformed for the better after they became aware of the benefits of psyllium and began incorporating it into their daily routine. One can say that this is an extremely satisfying experience.

I've realized that it's not just about sharing information; it's also about assisting other people on their own journey rather than just passing on information. The concepts of empathy, understanding, and support are essential. Every individual is one of a kind and faces their own set of peculiar obstacles to conquer. I want to assist them in locating the appropriate tools and resources so that they can accomplish their health objectives.

In the following section, I will discuss my experiences and insights with the purpose of motivating others and providing them with useful advice and direction. In addition to educating them on the significance of maintaining a healthy diet and using natural remedies such as psyllium, I want to assist them in making a decision that is beneficial to their health.

We are able to establish a movement of support and knowledge when we work together. I am convinced that each and every one of us possesses the capacity to enhance our health and to lead lives that are rich in happiness. Through the dissemination of my expertise and experiences, I hope to inspire others to embark on their own independent journeys and take responsibility for their own health.

Sharing the information that I have learned about psyllium and healthy eating is a gift that I take great pleasure in giving. One of my goals is to assist other people in improving their health, boosting their energy levels, and living a life that is rich in joy and vitality. Let us embark on a journey together to discover the world of health and assist others in undergoing their own personal transformation.

A sustainable change

Following the realization that psyllium was the key to my salvation, it was of utmost significance for me to incorporate this change into my life over the course of a longer period of time. In addition to the importance of finding short-term solutions, it is also essential to strive to maintain a lifestyle that is both sustainable and healthy.

The incorporation of psyllium seeds into my diet eventually became habitual for me. I started incorporating them into my daily routine, whether it was in the form of psyllium porridge for breakfast or as an ingredient in healthy baked goods and smoothies. I found that I was reaping the benefits of these foods. I came to the realization very quickly that psyllium was not only a solution to the health issues that I was experiencing, but it also became an essential component of my overall well-being.

Over time, I became aware of the ways in which this healthy lifestyle impacted every aspect of my life. I experienced an increase in my energy levels, a normalization of my digestion, and an overall feeling of greater equilibrium and vitality. It was almost as if I had discovered the secret to living a life that was both healthy and happy.

The long-term viability of this change was something that I placed a lot of importance on. I wanted to make sure that my new way of life was not just a passing fad but rather a habit that would last for a long time. In order to prepare a wide variety of meals that included psyllium, I started becoming more knowledgeable about healthy eating and expanding my cooking skills.

Maintaining this course of action was not always an easy task. There were times when I was tempted to revert to my previous behaviors or to allow the commotion and activity of my daily life to exert an excessive amount of influence over me. Every time, however, I recalled how much my life had improved and how much I had already accomplished. I was amazed at how much I had accomplished. This provided me with the impetus to maintain my level of determination and to carry on with my healthy lifestyle.

After a number of years have passed since my initial experience with psyllium, I am pleased to report that I have finally found my way. Psyllium seeds have proved to be a dependable companion throughout my life, assisting me in the preservation of my health and the enhancement of my overall well-being. Not only are they a fad or a short-term solution, but they are also an indispensable component of my long-term strategy for maintaining my health.

In this part of the article, I would like to talk about my experiences and encourage other people to work toward making changes that are sustainable as well. A healthy lifestyle is about realizing the long-term benefits of a healthy lifestyle, making conscious choices, and motivating yourself to live a healthy lifestyle. Psyllium, when combined with a diet that is well-balanced, has the potential to improve our long-term health and allow us to live a life that is rich in happiness.

It is not an easy path to change that is long-lasting, but it is one that is worth taking. Dedication, perseverance, and a willingness to push yourself to your limits are all necessary components. The payoff, however, is a life that is rich in vitality, health, and unending happiness. Join me on this adventure, and let's take pleasure in and rejoice in the transformations that we encounter along the way.

Conclusion

Within the context of this narrative of optimism and metamorphosis, I have shared my personal experience with psyllium, which has had a profound impact on my life. This has been a journey that has been full of difficulties, but it has also been full of favorable changes and rewards. By including psyllium in my diet, I was able to get rid of the digestive issues I had been experiencing, boost my energy levels, and reach a new level of wellness.

For as long as I can remember, my objective has been to inspire and motivate other people. In light of the fact that psyllium has made a significant difference in my life, I am confident that other people can also reap the benefits of its positive effects on their health. As a result, I strongly recommend that you embark on your own journey toward a life that is both healthy and happy.

To get started, you should begin by gathering information about psyllium and balanced eating. Numerous resources, books, and specialists are available to assist you in this endeavor. Make it a priority to educate yourself on the advantages of psyllium and the ways in which you can incorporate it into your diet. Have a willingness to change and be open to the idea of forming new routines.

I am aware that it is not always simple to break old habits and replace them with new ones without any difficulty. Both physical endurance and the willingness to step outside of one's comfort zone are required for this. But I can guarantee that it will be well worth it. It is impossible to overstate the importance of the positive change that you will experience.

Always keep in mind that everyone is on their own journey, and that it is not about excelling in everything. If you want to live a healthy life, even the smallest steps count. Exert patience with yourself and rejoice in every achievement, no matter how insignificant it may seem. When it comes to improving your health and happiness, each day presents a fresh opportunity.

In addition to that, I would like to provide you with some recommendations and resources of additional information. Make use of them to broaden your worldview and provide support for your journey. There are a variety of resources that can be helpful in expanding your knowledge of psyllium and healthy eating, including books, websites, and experts.

In conclusion, I would like to convey to you that you are deserving of living a life that is both healthy and happy. Maintain a positive attitude and keep in mind that transformation is attainable. Today is the day to begin writing your own personal story of transformation. On your path to living a life that is rich in meaning and vitality, I hope that you find success.

Greetings and best wishes, Within the context of this narrative of optimism and metamorphosis, I have shared my personal experience with psyllium, which has had a profound impact on my life. This has been a journey that has been full of difficulties, but it has also been full of favorable changes and rewards. By including psyllium in my diet, I was able to get rid of the digestive issues I had been experiencing, boost my energy levels, and reach a new level of wellness.

For as long as I can remember, my objective has been to inspire and motivate other people. In light of the fact that psyllium has made a significant difference in my life, I am confident that other people can also reap the benefits of its positive effects on their health. As a result, I strongly recommend that you embark on your own journey toward a life that is both healthy and happy.

To get started, you should begin by gathering information about psyllium and balanced eating. Numerous resources, books, and specialists are available to assist you in this endeavor. Make it a priority to educate yourself on the advantages of psyllium and the ways in which you can incorporate it into your diet. Have a willingness to change and be open to the idea of forming new routines.

I am aware that it is not always simple to break old habits and replace them with new ones without any difficulty. Both physical endurance and the willingness to step outside of one's comfort zone are required for this. But I can guarantee that it will be well worth it. It is impossible to overstate the importance of the positive change that you will experience.

Always keep in mind that everyone is on their own journey, and that it is not about excelling in everything. If you want to live a healthy life, even the smallest steps count. Exert patience with yourself and rejoice in every achievement, no matter how insignificant it may seem. When it comes to improving your health and happiness, each day presents a fresh opportunity.

In addition to that, I would like to provide you with some recommendations and resources of additional information. Make use of them to broaden your worldview and provide support for your journey. There are a variety of resources that can be helpful in expanding your knowledge of psyllium and healthy eating, including books, websites, and experts.

In conclusion, I would like to convey to you that you are deserving of living a life that is both healthy and happy. Maintain a positive attitude and keep in mind that transformation is attainable. Today is the day to begin writing your own personal story of transformation. On your path to living a life that is rich in meaning and vitality, I hope that you find success.

Greetings and best wishes,

Anna Miller

Psyllium: The natural source for health and well-being

Introduction

We would like to take this opportunity to welcome you to our exciting journey into the world of psyllium seeds, which are a natural source of health and wellness. The purpose of this article is to provide you with an introduction to the fundamentals of incorporating psyllium seeds into your diet and to assist you in comprehending the remarkable advantages that these tiny seeds offer. You will find all of the information that you require to delve into this subject, regardless of whether or not you are familiar with the term "psyllium."

You might be wondering why, of all things, psyllium would be chosen. Why should we bother with them, and what is it about them that makes them so unique? Psyllium seeds, on the other hand, are not a recently discovered superfood that has been gaining popularity; rather, they have a long history and have been valued for their health benefits for centuries. Despite the fact that they were originally indigenous to India, psyllium seeds have gained popularity as a dietary supplement in other regions of the world as well. However, what exactly is it that sets them apart from other people?

But before we get into the specifics, let's take a quick look at the history of psyllium seeds and where they came from. India, the Mediterranean region, and certain regions of North America are the primary locations where the plantago ovata plant is cultivated. These small seeds originate from this plant. In traditional medicine, psyllium seeds have been used for a variety of purposes, particularly to aid digestion and general well-being, for a number of generations.

Because of its ability to bind water and form a substance that is similar to gel, psyllium is an extremely exciting substance to use. They expand and form a protective layer that helps digestion while also assisting in the regulation of bowel movements when they come into contact with liquid. People who struggle with digestive issues, such as constipation or irritable bowel syndrome, can benefit from psyllium because it is a natural solution to these issues.

Incorporating psyllium seeds into your diet is a straightforward and uncomplicated process. It is simple to incorporate them into your daily routine, whether you choose to do so by incorporating them into smoothies, yogurt, or cereal, or even by utilizing them in recipes for baking. The adaptability of psyllium seeds enables you to incorporate them into your diet in a wide variety of ways, allowing you to take advantage of the numerous health benefits they offer.

Nevertheless, it is of utmost significance to keep in mind that when consuming psyllium seeds, it is essential to consume an adequate amount of fluids. Due to the fact that they have a high capacity for swelling, it is absolutely necessary for you to consume a sufficient amount of water or other liquids in order to optimize digestion and prevent any potential blockages.

We are going to delve deeper into the health benefits of psyllium in the following sections. These benefits include an aid to digestion, the regulation of cholesterol levels, and the promotion of a feeling of fullness that lasts for a long time. In addition to this, you will receive useful advice and recommendations on how to incorporate psyllium into your daily routine so that you can reap the benefits of these positive experiences.

You are prepared to enter the realm of psyllium, are you? Let us spend some time together investigating the fundamentals and learning about the incredible opportunities they present for our health and well-being. Whether you are looking for natural solutions to your digestive issues or simply want to improve your lifestyle in general, psyllium might be exactly what you have been looking for all along.

Investigate psyllium seeds and gain a better understanding of their applications as well as the remarkable advantages they offer to each and every one of us. Collectively, we will investigate the ways in which psyllium seeds can assist us in our pursuit of a life that is both healthy and fulfilling.

Please be aware that the information contained in this text is not meant to serve as a replacement for the advice of a medical professional. Please seek the advice of a qualified medical professional or nutritionist if you have any concerns or questions regarding the use of psyllium that are specific to your health situations.We would like to take this opportunity to welcome you to our exciting journey into the world of psyllium seeds, which are a natural source of health and wellness. The purpose of this article is to provide you with an introduction to the fundamentals of incorporating psyllium seeds into your diet and to assist you in comprehending the remarkable advantages that these tiny seeds offer. You will find all of the information that you require to delve into this subject, regardless of whether or not you are familiar with the term "psyllium."

You might be wondering why, of all things, psyllium would be chosen. Why should we bother with them, and what is it about them that makes them so unique? Psyllium seeds, on the other hand, are not a recently discovered superfood that has been gaining popularity; rather, they have a long history and have been valued for their health benefits for centuries. Despite the fact that they were originally indigenous to India, psyllium seeds have gained popularity as a dietary supplement in other regions of the world as well. However, what exactly is it that sets them apart from other people?

But before we get into the specifics, let's take a quick look at the history of psyllium seeds and where they came from. India, the Mediterranean region, and certain regions of North America are the primary locations where the plantago ovata plant is cultivated. These small seeds originate from this plant. In traditional medicine, psyllium seeds have been used for a variety of purposes, particularly to aid digestion and general well-being, for a number of generations.

Because of its ability to bind water and form a substance that is similar to gel, psyllium is an extremely exciting substance to use. They expand and form a protective layer that helps digestion while also assisting in the regulation of bowel movements when they come into contact with liquid. People who struggle with digestive issues, such as constipation or irritable bowel syndrome, can benefit from psyllium because it is a natural solution to these issues.

Incorporating psyllium seeds into your diet is a straightforward and uncomplicated process. It is simple to incorporate them into your daily routine, whether you choose to do so by incorporating them into smoothies, yogurt, or cereal, or even by utilizing them in recipes for baking. The adaptability of psyllium seeds enables you to incorporate them into your diet in a wide variety of ways, allowing you to take advantage of the numerous health benefits they offer.

Nevertheless, it is of utmost significance to keep in mind that when consuming psyllium seeds, it is essential to consume an adequate amount of fluids. Due to the fact that they have a high capacity for swelling, it is absolutely necessary for you to consume a sufficient amount of water or other liquids in order to optimize digestion and prevent any potential blockages.

We are going to delve deeper into the health benefits of psyllium in the following sections. These benefits include an aid to digestion, the regulation of cholesterol levels, and the promotion of a feeling of fullness that lasts for a long time. In addition to this, you will receive useful advice and recommendations on how to incorporate psyllium into your daily routine so that you can reap the benefits of these positive experiences.

You are prepared to enter the realm of psyllium, are you? Let us spend some time together investigating the fundamentals and learning about the incredible opportunities they present for our health and well-being. Whether you are looking for natural solutions to your digestive issues or simply want to improve your lifestyle in general, psyllium might be exactly what you have been looking for all along.

Investigate psyllium seeds and gain a better understanding of their applications as well as the remarkable advantages they offer to each and every one of us. Collectively, we will investigate the ways in which psyllium seeds can assist us in our pursuit of a life that is both healthy and fulfilling.

Please be aware that the information contained in this text is not meant to serve as a replacement for the advice of a medical professional. Please seek the advice of a qualified medical professional or nutritionist if you have any concerns or questions regarding the use of psyllium that are specific to your health situations.

Chapter 1: The health benefits of psyllium

1.1 Promotion of healthy digestion

It is essential to our overall health that we have a healthy digestive system. On the other hand, irregularities can occasionally take place, which can put a strain on our bodies. The psyllium seeds come into play at this point in the process. They are able to promote healthy digestion due to the presence of soluble fiber, which is a unique component of their composition.

Imagine that you have been experiencing discomfort and that you have been struggling with constipation for several days. This is quite frustrating and can have a significant impact on your day-to-day life. Taking psyllium seeds, on the other hand, can provide you with a natural source of relief. The fiber in the seeds forms a gel-like substance in the digestive tract, where it binds water and causes it to pass through. This causes the stool to become more pliable, which makes it easier for it to move through the intestines. Consuming psyllium seeds on a consistent basis can assist in the prevention of constipation and the promotion of smooth digestion.

1.2 Relief from constipation

Constipation can result in a wide range of associated symptoms. It is unpleasant to experience the effects, which include a feeling of bloating, pain, and discomfort. If you have ever suffered from constipation, you are aware of how critical it is to locate a remedy for the condition.

If you want to get your digestion going again, psyllium seeds can be of assistance. Stool volume is increased and bowel movement is stimulated as a result of the fiber found in the seeds. Constipation is alleviated and bowel movements are made easier as a result of this. A great number of individuals have reported favorable outcomes as a result of incorporating psyllium seeds into their diet. They have reported experiencing noticeably improved quality of life as well as relief.

1.3 Support for intestinal health

What determines our overall health is the condition of our intestines. It is an essential component in the process of absorbing nutrients and enhancing the capability of our immune system. However, there are times when the equilibrium of the intestinal flora can be disrupted, which can result in discomfort and a general feeling of unwellness.

Seeds of psyllium have been shown to be beneficial to intestinal health. The seeds contain soluble fiber, which acts as a source of nourishment for the beneficial bacteria that live in the intestines. This helps to restore balance and encourages the growth of healthy intestinal flora throughout the body. When it comes to optimal digestion, the absorption of nutrients, and protection against inflammatory diseases in the digestive tract, having a balanced intestinal flora is one of the most important factors.

1.4 Reduction of gastrointestinal complaints

The symptoms of flatulence, irritable bowel syndrome, and acid regurgitation are also associated with the gastrointestinal tract and are experienced by a significant number of individuals. It is possible for these complaints to significantly impair one's overall well-being and to place a strain on day-to-day life.

Psyllium seeds are another source of extremely helpful support in this regard. By acting as a protective barrier on the mucosa of the gastrointestinal tract, the gel-like substance that is produced as a result of the swelling of the seeds has the potential to alleviate the symptoms of these complaints. After consuming psyllium seeds on a consistent basis, a number of individuals have reported experiencing a discernible improvement in their symptoms as well as relief in the gastrointestinal tract.

Psyllium seeds are a natural remedy that can be used to treat a variety of digestive issues. Relieving constipation, promoting healthy digestion, supporting intestinal health, and reducing gastrointestinal discomfort are all benefits of using them. You are able to provide your body with natural support and achieve a higher level of health and wellness if you include psyllium seeds in your diet. Throughout the subsequent chapters, we will delve into additional fascinating aspects of psyllium and demonstrate how you can incorporate it into your diet in order to reap the numerous advantages that it offers.

Chapter 2: Weight management with psyllium

2.1 Appetite-suppressing properties of psyllium seeds

The ability to exercise control over one's appetite is an essential component of effective weight management. Consuming an excessive amount of food and maintaining control over one's eating habits are challenges that many people face. In this regard, psyllium seeds have the potential to offer beneficial support.

For some reason, psyllium seeds have the remarkable ability to cause the stomach to expand, which in turn results in a feeling of fullness. It is possible for psyllium seeds to form a gel-like mass in the stomach if they are consumed prior to a meal and if they are done so with sufficient water. A volume is produced as a result of this, which contributes to the feeling of satiety and helps to fill the stomach. This may result in you eating less food, which will allow you to better control your appetite.

Regarding its effectiveness as an appetite suppressant, psyllium has been praised by a great number of individuals. Individuals who have taken psyllium have reported that it makes them feel fuller more quickly and reduces their desire for unhealthy snacks and foods. You will be able to support your efforts to manage your weight and make it easier to combat unhealthy eating habits if you include psyllium in your diet.

2.2 Support for weight reduction

It is essential to combine a diet that is both healthy and balanced with regular physical activity in order to achieve the goal of losing certain amount of weight. It is possible that psyllium will be an advantageous addition to support your goals.

Additionally, the fiber that is found in psyllium has the capacity to bind water and produce volume. This results in a longer feeling of satiety and can assist in reducing the desire to consume food. Furthermore, the fiber helps to maintain healthy digestion and regulates blood sugar levels, both of which are essential for maintaining a stable energy balance and increasing the ability to exercise better control over eating behavior.

On the other hand, it is essential to stress that psyllium seeds by themselves do not magically restore health. They ought to be consumed as a component of a diet that is both well-balanced and mindful of calorie intake. In order to achieve a well-rounded meal, you should combine them with fresh fruits and vegetables, lean protein, and healthy fats respectively. It is also recommended that you make regular exercise a part of your daily routine in order to support your efforts to lose weight.

2.3 Psyllium as part of a balanced diet

Not only are psyllium seeds an effective tool for weight loss, but they are also an essential component of a diet that is both healthy and well-balanced. Additionally, they are a source of fiber, which not only helps maintain a healthy weight but also promotes healthy digestion.

Consuming an adequate amount of fiber is essential for maintaining overall health because fiber promotes intestinal health and can assist in the prevention of constipation. They promote the formation of healthy intestinal flora and improve blood circulation in the digestive tract, which is essential for proper digestion.

If you include psyllium in your diet, you will be able to increase the amount of fiber you consume, which will also enhance the beneficial effects that fiber has on your digestion and your ability to control your weight. In order to give your body time to adjust, you should begin with a small amount and gradually increase it.

A number of different ways are available for you to incorporate psyllium seeds into your diet. For instance, you can incorporate them into frozen yogurt, cereals, or smoothies; you can also use them as a binder in soups and sauces; and you can use them in baked goods. Psyllium seeds can be utilized in a variety of inventive ways, and the health benefits they offer can be maximized.

Within the scope of this chapter, we have underscored the significance of psyllium in the context of weight management. Their ability to suppress appetite, in addition to their function as an integral component of a well-balanced diet, can assist you in reaching your desired weight. In the following chapter, we will discuss yet another significant aspect, which is the role that psyllium plays in maintaining healthy cholesterol levels.

Chapter 3: Cardiovascular Health and Psyllium

3.1 Lowering the cholesterol level

It is of utmost significance for the health of the cardiovascular system to keep cholesterol levels at a healthy level. A higher cholesterol level can make the risk of developing heart disease higher. Because it has the ability to reduce cholesterol levels, psyllium is a useful supplement in this regard.

There is a specific kind of dietary fiber known as soluble fiber that can be found in psyllium. When these soluble fibers come into contact with water in the intestine, they are able to combine and produce a substance that is similar to a gel. This substance helps to eliminate bile acids from the body by binding to them in the intestines and facilitating their elimination. Since bile acids are produced from cholesterol, an increase in the excretion of bile acids can result in a reduction in the levels of cholesterol found in the body.

There have been numerous studies that have demonstrated that taking psyllium can result in a significant reduction in LDL cholesterol, which is also referred to as "bad" cholesterol. A decrease in LDL cholesterol is associated with a reduction in the risk of cardiovascular disease and the hardening of the arteries.

An illustration of this would be Mrs. Muller, who consisted of psyllium in her diet on a consistent basis. After taking psyllium and adhering to a healthy diet for a period of several months, she noticed a significant decrease in the levels of LDL cholesterol they contained. It was confirmed by her physician that the incorporation of psyllium can be an effective measure to improve cardiovascular health. Her physician was impressed by the results.

3.2 Blood pressure regulation and protection against heart disease

Blood pressure regulation is another essential component of cardiovascular health that must be taken into consideration. If you have high blood pressure, also referred to as hypertension, you may be at an increased risk of developing heart disease. Psyllium has been shown to have a natural ability to regulate blood pressure and to lower the risk of developing heart disease.

Because it helps to support the vascular system, the soluble fiber that is found in psyllium can assist in lowering blood pressure. Both the blood vessels and the blood circulation are improved as a result of their relaxing effect on the blood vessels. Blood pressure is lowered as a result of this because the pressure on the vessel walls is reduced.

According to the findings of one study, patients with mild to moderate hypertension who consumed psyllium on a regular basis experienced a significant reduction in their cardiovascular blood pressure. According to these findings, psyllium has the potential to be an effective supplement for the management of blood pressure.Blood pressure regulation is another essential component of cardiovascular health that must be taken into consideration. If you have high blood pressure, also referred to as hypertension, you may be at an increased risk of developing heart disease. Psyllium has been shown to have a natural ability to regulate blood pressure and to lower the risk of developing heart disease.

Because it helps to support the vascular system, the soluble fiber that is found in psyllium can assist in lowering blood pressure. Both the blood vessels and the blood circulation are improved as a result of their relaxing effect on the blood vessels. Blood pressure is lowered as a result of this because the pressure on the vessel walls is reduced.

According to the findings of one study, patients with mild to moderate hypertension who consumed psyllium on a regular basis experienced a significant reduction in their cardiovascular blood pressure. According to these findings, psyllium has the potential to be an effective supplement for the management of blood pressure.

3.3 Anti-inflammatory effect of psyllium

The development of cardiovascular disease is significantly influenced by inflammation as a key factor. Inflammation that is chronic in the body can lead to damage to the blood vessels, which in turn raises the risk of cardiovascular events like heart attacks and strokes. It is possible that the anti-inflammatory properties of psyllium can assist in the reduction of inflammation.

The soluble fiber found in psyllium has the ability to prevent the growth of certain bacteria that are known to cause inflammation in the intestines. Psyllium helps promote healthy intestinal flora and reduces the risk of inflammation by limiting the growth of these bacteria, which in turn helps to preserve intestinal health.

Additionally, psyllium is a source of antioxidants, which have the ability to counteract the effects of free radicals in the body. Molecular substances known as free radicals have the potential to cause inflammation within the body. Psyllium has the ability to reduce inflammation in the body because it prevents the formation of free radicals.

An example that is more concrete is Mr. Schmidt, who has been incorporating psyllium into his diet on a consistent basis. Earlier in his life, he had been experiencing persistent inflammation throughout his body, which had a negative impact on his cardiovascular health. He noticed a significant improvement in his inflammation levels and felt better overall after taking psyllium for a few months. He also noticed that his overall health had improved.

Our research in this chapter has focused on the effects that psyllium has on the health of the cardiovascular system. As a result of its ability to reduce cholesterol levels, regulate blood pressure, and have an anti-inflammatory effect, psyllium has the potential to make a significant contribution to the maintenance of a physically healthy cardiovascular system. In the following chapter, we will discuss another facet, which is the supportive role that psyllium plays for the immune system.

Chapter 4: Diabetes management with psyllium

4.1 Effects of psyllium on blood glucose levels

Diabetes, also known as simply diabetes, is a metabolic disease that is characterized by elevated blood sugar levels. Seeds of psyllium have the potential to offer natural assistance in the regulation of blood sugar levels. A significant part of this process is played by the soluble dietary fiber that they consume.

Consuming food causes the carbohydrates that are present in the food to be converted into glucose, which in turn causes an increase in the amount of glucose that is within the blood. On the other hand, the synthesis of glucose in the intestine is slowed down by the presence of soluble fiber in psyllium. Because of this, there is no sudden increase in the levels of glucose in the blood, and the rise is slower and more consistent. When it comes to maintaining stable blood glucose levels, this is especially helpful for people who have diabetes because it helps them remain stable.

An illustration of this would be Mrs. Schneider, who is afflicted with type 2 diabetes. She observed an improvement in her ability to maintain control of her blood sugar levels after she began including psyllium in her diet. After taking the medication, she was able to observe that her blood glucose levels had become more stable, with fewer spikes and lows. Because of this, she was able to better control her diabetes, which in turn helped her reduce the amount of insulin she required.

4.2 Improvement of insulin resistance

Insulin resistance is a condition that occurs when cells in the body no longer respond appropriately to insulin, which is the hormone that controls the amount of sugar that is present in the blood. This is one of the characteristics that is associated with type 2 diabetes. Increasing the sensitivity of cells to insulin and lowering insulin resistance are both possible benefits of psyllium utilization.

Psyllium contains soluble fiber, which has the potential to improve the rate at which glucose is absorbed into cells. They accomplish this by reducing the rate of digestion, which gives cells more time to react to insulin and improves the efficiency with which they absorb glucose. This contributes to a reduction in insulin resistance as well as a decrease in blood glucose levels.

There is a good illustration of this in Mr. Muller. Insulin resistance was a symptom of his type 2 diabetes, which he was diagnosed with some time ago. The gradual improvement in his insulin resistance that he observed after incorporating psyllium into his diet was a result of his efforts. His blood glucose levels eventually became more stable, and his physician was able to observe a decrease in the amount of insulin that he was taking.

4.3 Psyllium as a support for diabetes control

When it comes to managing diabetes, psyllium seeds can be an extremely helpful addition. It is important to note that in addition to regulating blood sugar levels and improving insulin resistance, they also provide additional benefits to individuals who have diabetes.

As a result of the high fiber content that they contain, psyllium seeds have the ability to help increase feelings of satiety and also reduce cravings. Due to the fact that maintaining a healthy weight and eating a balanced diet are both essential components of diabetes management, this can be of particular assistance.

There is also the possibility that psyllium can assist in lowering cholesterol, which is an additional concern for a lot of people who have diabetes. The risk of cardiovascular disease, which is already elevated in people who have diabetes, can be increased by having high cholesterol levels.

Psyllium seeds, in general, should be considered a valuable support for people who have diabetes because they can assist in the regulation of blood sugar levels, the improvement of insulin resistance, and the promotion of a healthy diet. However, it is essential to clarify that psyllium seeds are not intended to serve as a replacement for conventional medical treatment. Before making any adjustments to their method of treatment or diet, individuals who have diabetes should always discuss their options with their primary care physician.

Through the consumption of psyllium, we will investigate yet another significant subject in the following chapter: the promotion of healthy digestion and the prevention of digestive problems.

Chapter 5: Psyllium for healthy intestinal flora

5.1 Prebiotic properties of psyllium seeds

The intestinal flora that is in good health is an important factor in our overall health and well-being. Due to the presence of prebiotic properties, psyllium seeds can be beneficial in assisting in the maintenance of a healthy intestinal flora. Prebiotics are components of food that encourage the growth and activity of beneficial bacteria in the intestines because they are bioactive.

The soluble fiber found in psyllium provides nourishment for the beneficial bacteria that are present in the body, particularly the types of bacteria that are essential for maintaining a healthy intestinal flora. Psyllium helps promote the growth and proliferation of beneficial bacteria by providing nourishment to these bacteria. This helps to maintain the healthy balance of intestinal flora and prevents the growth of bacteria that are harmful to the body.

In this regard, Mrs. Schmidt is a good example because she frequently struggled with digestive issues. As a result of incorporating psyllium into her diet, she experienced a reduction in abdominal pain and bloating, as well as an improvement in her digestion. This was attributed to the prebiotic properties of psyllium, which assisted in rebalancing the flora that was present in her intestinal tract.

5.2 Promoting the growth of good intestinal bacteria

Psyllium has the ability to not only encourage the growth of beneficial bacteria in the intestines but also to boost the activity of those bacteria. Beneficial bacteria are responsible for the production of short-chain fatty acids, which are an essential component in the process of preserving intestinal health. Additionally, these fatty acids contribute to the maintenance of a healthy intestinal mucosa by acting as a source of energy for the cells that make up the colon.

With its ability to encourage the growth and activity of beneficial bacteria, psyllium contributes to an increase in the production of short-chain fatty acids. The inflammation in the gut can be reduced, nutrient absorption can be improved, and overall gut health can be supported while doing this.

Additionally, Mr. Wagner had a disturbed intestinal flora, which contributed to his chronic intestinal problems. As a result of his consistent consumption of psyllium, he observed a notable improvement in the digestive symptoms he was experiencing. The bloating he experienced was reduced, and he experienced fewer instances of constipation. This resulted in an overall enhanced sense of well-being as well as an improvement in the quality of life.

5.3 Effects on the immune system and general health

Not only does a healthy intestinal flora play a significant part in digestion, but it also has an effect on the immune system and an individual's overall health. When it comes to protecting ourselves from illness, having a healthy immune system is absolutely necessary.

By promoting the growth of beneficial intestinal flora, psyllium has the ability to fortify the immune system and contribute to the reduction of inflammation throughout the body. As a result, this may have a beneficial impact on the prevention of diseases and on overall health.

An illustration of this would be Mrs. Muller, who had to contend with colds and infections on a regular basis. Following the incorporation of psyllium into her diet, she observed a notable enhancement in the effectiveness of her immune defense function. In general, she felt more energized and vital, and she experienced fewer instances of illness.

Because of its prebiotic properties, the fact that it encourages the growth of beneficial bacteria, and the effects that it has on the immune system, psyllium is an extremely valuable natural source for promoting normal intestinal flora. When we include psyllium in our diet, we are able to improve the health of our intestinal tract, reduce the severity of digestive issues, and enhance our overall well-being.

We will discuss yet another significant subject in the following chapter, which is the numerous ways in which psyllium can be utilized to contribute to a healthy diet.

Chapter 6: Detoxification and cleansing of the body with psyllium

6.1 The ability of psyllium to bind and eliminate toxins

Psyllium seeds have the remarkable ability to bind and eliminate toxins from the body, which is one of the many impressive properties of these seeds. As a result of their gel-like consistency, psyllium seeds have the ability to absorb harmful substances in the digestive tract whenever they come into contact with water. This allows them to naturally eliminate these substances from the body.

Mr. Mayer is a good example of someone who uses psyllium as part of a cleansing treatment on a regular basis. He experiences a general sense of lightness, improved digestion, and increased energy while he is receiving treatment for his condition. It is his firm belief that the detoxifying properties of psyllium assist in the elimination of harmful substances from his bloodstream.

6.2 Reduction of pollutants in the body

Pollution, the presence of pesticides in food, and the consumption of processed goods are all examples of ways in which we are constantly exposed to potentially hazardous substances in our contemporary world. These contaminants have the potential to build up in the body, which can result in a variety of health issues.

Psyllium seeds have the potential to lessen the impact that is caused by pollutants in the body. Psyllium does this by binding toxins and removing them from the digestive tract. This helps reduce the amount of harmful substances that are absorbed by the body and deposited in the tissues.

Over the course of her life, Ms. Schneider had been dealing with skin issues, which she believed were caused by her prolonged exposure to environmental toxins. Her skin health began to improve after she started including psyllium in her diet, and she noticed this improvement straight away. Her skin became more radiant and clear, which she attributed to the decreased exposure to pollutants in her body. She also noticed that her skin became clearer.

6.3 Psyllium as a natural detox method

When it comes to detoxifying the body, psyllium seeds are a method that is both natural and gentle. When compared to radical diets or aggressive detoxification programs, psyllium seeds are able to assist the body in removing harmful substances in a soft and gentle manner.

Psyllium seeds are beneficial to the natural detoxification process of the body because they help to cleanse the intestines and ensure that bowel movements are regular. In addition to protecting the health of the intestinal tract, they facilitate the efficient elimination of waste and toxins.

Ms. Schmidt is overjoyed with the results of her psyllium detox regimen, which she has been strictly adhering to on a consistent basis. She reports enhancements in the appearance of her skin, an increase in her energy levels, and an overall sense of well-being. When it comes to regularly detoxifying and cleansing her body, she finds that psyllium seeds are an effective and natural method.

As a result of its detoxifying properties, psyllium is an extremely useful natural source for ridding the body of potentially harmful substances. By including psyllium in our diet, we are able to provide our body with support in a way that is both gentle and effective, thereby achieving a state of well-being that is both healthy and vital.

Within the following chapter, we will discuss the practical aspects of utilizing psyllium, as well as provide you with some suggestions and recommendations on how to incorporate psyllium into your daily routine in order to reap the numerous health benefits that it offers.

Chapter 7: Skin health and psyllium

7.1 Effects of psyllium on the skin

There is evidence that psyllium seeds not only have beneficial effects on digestion and the internal organs of the body, but they also have the potential to significantly influence the health of our skin. They have the ability to help improve the texture of the skin and promote a radiant complexion due to the natural properties and nutrients that they contain.

One young woman named Lisa, who had been battling acne for a number of years, is a remarkable illustration of this phenomenon. She began to observe a gradual but noticeable improvement in the condition of her skin after she began including psyllium in her overall diet. While the cleansing action of psyllium assisted in the removal of excess oil and impurities, the anti-inflammatory properties of psyllium helped reduce redness and swelling.

7.2 Alleviation of skin problems such as acne and eczema.

Furthermore, psyllium seeds have the potential to offer significant assistance in the treatment of skin conditions such as acne and eczema. Because of their anti-inflammatory properties and their capacity to eliminate toxins from the body, psyllium seeds have the potential to assist in the reduction of skin irritation and the acceleration of the healing pathway.

Mr. Muller had been battling eczema for many years, which caused his skin to become extremely itchy and irritated. Following the beginning of his consumption of psyllium, he observed a notable improvement in the symptoms he was experiencing. The naturally occurring substances found in psyllium helped reduce inflammation and relieve itching, which ultimately resulted in skin that appeared to be healthier and more soothed.

7.3 Beauty benefits of psyllium for healthy skin and hair

Furthermore, psyllium has the potential to not only alleviate skin problems but also contribute to the development of more beautiful skin and healthier hair. Their abundant nutritional composition, which includes omega-3 fatty acids and antioxidants, helps to promote the production of collagen, enhances the elasticity of the skin, and fortifies the hair from the inside out.

Brittle hair, which broke easily and appeared dull, was a problem that Mrs. Wagner had struggled with for her entire life. Following the incorporation of psyllium into her diet, she observed that her hair gradually became more robust and healthy than before. Her explanation was that the nutrient-rich properties of psyllium were responsible for the increased shine and volume that it exhibited.

In light of this, psyllium has the potential to not only contribute to the maintenance of a healthy digestive system and overall well-being, but it can also support the health and beauty of our skin and hair.

In the following chapter, we will discuss the practical applications of psyllium in the kitchen. We will also provide you with some ideas for innovative recipes and helpful hints on how to incorporate psyllium into your meals so that you can reap the benefits of all of these qualities.

Chapter 8: Psyllium in children's nutrition

8.1 Safety and dosage of psyllium for children

If we are concerned about the health of our children, it is essential that we make certain that they are receiving the appropriate substances. The addition of psyllium to a child's diet can be beneficial; however, it is essential to ensure that the appropriate dosage and safety measures are followed.

According to the child's age and weight, the appropriate dosage of psyllium should be determined. In order to acclimate the body to the fiber, it is recommended to begin with a low dosage and gradually increase it over time. In order to ensure that the dosage is appropriate for your child, it is recommended that you consult with a nutritionist or a pediatrician before making any decisions regarding the dosage.

8.2 Benefits of psyllium for children's digestion

The consumption of psyllium seeds can have a beneficial impact on the digestive system of children and assist them in maintaining healthy bowel function. When it comes to the absorption of nutrients and the prevention of digestive issues like constipation, having a healthy digestive system is absolutely necessary.

Tom, an eight-year-old boy, is a good example of someone who frequently experienced digestive issues and difficulties with constipation. As soon as his parents started including psyllium in his diet, they observed a significant improvement in the state of his digestive health. Due to the presence of fiber in psyllium, regular bowel movements were encouraged, and elimination was made easier, which ultimately simplified digestion.

8.3 Integration of psyllium in child-friendly recipes

The process of incorporating psyllium into the diets of children presents a number of challenges, one of which is the search for kid-friendly recipes that cater to the preferences and tastes of young children. The following are some suggestions for incorporating psyllium into the meals that your children consume:

You can incorporate psyllium seeds into smoothies by incorporating a small quantity of psyllium seeds into the smoothie that your child enjoys the most. The smooth consistency of the smoothie will make it simple to consume the seeds without any difficulty.

Psyllium seeds can be used as an alternative to eggs in baking recipes. Psyllium seeds can be used in place of eggs in baking recipes. For the purpose of achieving a fluffy consistency and binding the dough, a mixture of ground psyllium and water can be utilized successfully.

Sprinkle psyllium over breakfast cereal or yogurt: If you want to make it simple for your children to consume psyllium, you can do so by simply sprinkling it over their preferred breakfast cereal or yogurt. Extra fiber and nutrients are added to meals as a result of this.

You can ensure that your children will reap the health benefits of this natural source of health and wellness by incorporating psyllium into their diet in this manner. At the same time, you can ensure that they will enjoy delicious meals that are suitable for children.

Keep in mind that the introduction of new foods into your child's diet should be done in a slow and gradual manner, and you should be on the lookout for any suspected allergic reactions. If you have any questions or concerns, you should always seek the advice of a pediatrician or dietitian in order to determine the most appropriate course of action for your child.

Therefore, psyllium can be an advantageous addition to the diets of children in order to better support the health of their digestive systems and to incorporate the advantages of fiber into their diets.

Chapter 9: Tips for using psyllium in the kitchen

9.1 Different ways of using psyllium in recipes

Because of their high degree of adaptability, psyllium seeds can be utilized in a wide variety of culinary applications. You can incorporate psyllium seeds into your cooking in a variety of ways, including the following:

Using psyllium seeds as a thickener in sauces and soups is a natural alternative to using starch or flour. If you are looking for a natural alternative to these two ingredients, you can use psyllium seeds. Your dishes will have a more satisfying texture as a result of the seeds' ability to absorb liquid and give them a gel-like consistency.

In the realm of baked goods, psyllium seeds have the potential to function as an alternative to eggs or fat in baking recipes. It is possible to use psyllium seeds that have been ground in conjunction with water as a binder. The use of this is especially helpful for individuals who are allergic to eggs or fats, as well as for those who are interested in making their baked goods healthier.

Psyllium seeds can also be added to smoothies and drinks in order to increase the amount of fiber that is contained in these beverages. If you want a smoother texture, you can either use whole psyllium seeds or grind them before going through the process.

9.2 Cooking and preparation tips for optimal use of the benefits of psyllium.

It is essential to cook and prepare psyllium in the appropriate manner in order to realize its full potential benefits. I have some advice that will be of assistance to you:

It is possible to improve the gelling ability of psyllium seeds by soaking them before using them with other ingredients. After placing the seeds in a bowl of water, allow them to soak for a minimum of ten to fifteen minutes. Because of this, they are simpler to digest, and the body is able to absorb their fiber more effectively that way.

When consuming psyllium seeds, it is essential to ensure that you are staying hydrated by drinking an adequate amount of liquid. In the digestive tract, the seeds are able to absorb water and can cause swelling. They have the potential to cause constipation if there is not enough fluid present. When consuming psyllium seeds, it is imperative that you drink an adequate amount of water.

Psyllium seeds should be stored in a container that is airtight and placed in a cool and dry location in order to maintain their quality and freshness before being consumed. As an additional method for extending the shelf life of ground psyllium seeds, you can also store them in the refrigerator.

9.3 Creative ideas for incorporating psyllium into the daily diet

There are a lot of inventive ways to include psyllium in your diet on a regular basis and still reap the benefits of doing so for your health. I have some suggestions for you to consider:

In order to make psyllium pudding, combine ground psyllium seeds with the milk of your choice (for example, almond milk or oat milk), and then allow the mixture to sit for a few minutes until it begins to thicken. After that, you can enjoy a tantalizing psyllium pudding by adding some honey or fruit to it.

If you want to increase the amount of fiber in your cereal and feel fuller for a longer period of time, try adding a handful of psyllium to your bowl of cereal. As an additional option for a breakfast that is both nutritious and healthy, you can combine whole psyllium seeds with yogurt and fruit.

Homemade psyllium burgers can be made by using ground psyllium seeds as a binder in the hamburger mixture. They help to improve the texture of the burgers and maintain their juicy quality.

Crackers made with psyllium seeds can be made by combining ground psyllium seeds with spices and water to form a dough mixture. On a thin surface, roll out the dough, and then cut it into small squares. Psyllium crackers are a delicious and nutritious snack option that can be made by baking the squares in the oven until they reach a crispiest texture.

You can incorporate psyllium into your favorite recipes and reap the benefits of its health benefits by letting your imagination run wild and incorporating it for yourself. Discover new ways to incorporate psyllium into your diet by experimenting with a variety of preparation methods and finding new ways to incorporate it.

Conclusion

Psyllium, which is described as the natural source of health and well-being, provides a multitude of advantages for our health. Within the scope of this article, we have conducted an in-depth investigation into the numerous practical applications of psyllium seeds and the positive effects that they have on various parts of the body. Psyllium seeds offer a number of advantages, which can be summarized as follows:

Taking psyllium can assist in lowering cholesterol levels, which in turn can reduce the likelihood of developing cardiovascular disease. In addition to this, they assist in the regulation of blood pressure and offer protection against cardiovascular disease. Additionally, they possess anti-inflammatory properties, which mean that they can assist in the reduction of inflammation within the body.

Diabetes management is yet another area in which psyllium has been shown to have beneficial effects. In addition to enhancing insulin resistance, they have the ability to control blood sugar levels. When it comes to the management of diabetes, psyllium seeds can therefore be utilized as a nutritional supplement.

In addition, psyllium seeds are advantageous for maintaining a healthy flora in the intestinal tract. The prebiotic properties of these foods encourage the growth of beneficial bacteria in the intestines, which in turn helps to maintain healthy digestion. In addition to having beneficial effects on the immune system and overall health, a healthy intestinal flora is also beneficial.

The body can also be detoxified and cleansed with the help of psyllium seeds. As a result of their capacity to bind and eliminate toxins, they can contribute to the reduction of harmful substances that are found in the body. In the context of natural detoxification, they provide a gentle approach to the elimination of harmful substances from the body.

In addition, the use of psyllium is beneficial to the health of the skin. These products have the ability to alleviate skin conditions such as acne and eczema, and they also offer beauty benefits for maintaining healthy skin and hair.

However, in order to reap the full benefits of psyllium, it is essential to use it in the appropriate manner. Ensure that you consume the recommended dosage and that you drink an adequate amount of fluids while you are taking it. Additionally, psyllium ought to be incorporated into the diets of children, with safety and dosage considerations being taken into account.

To summarize, psyllium seeds are a natural source of health and well-being that many people find beneficial. Because of their versatility in the kitchen, they can be incorporated into daily diets in a diverse and inventive manner. Psyllium can be consumed in a wide variety of delicious forms, ranging from psyllium pudding and psyllium cereal to psyllium burgers and psyllium crackers, all of which are beneficial to nutritional health.

Psyllium and its effects on health are the subject of ongoing research, which is not standing still. If further research is conducted, it may be possible to gain additional insights into their mode of action and potential applications. It is important to keep a close eye on the upcoming developments in this field.

Psyllium seeds, in general, provide a method that is both natural and efficient for promoting positive health. They are an important component of a well-balanced diet because they offer numerous advantages, including the management of diabetes, the health of the intestinal flora, the detoxification process, the health of the skin, and many others. Now is the time to begin incorporating psyllium into your diet so that you can witness firsthand the positive effects that it has on your health and overall well-being.

Psyllium cuisine: healthy recipes for every meal

Introduction

Psyllium seeds are a wonderful addition to a healthy diet and can be used in many ways in cooking. They are rich in fiber and offer numerous health benefits. In this introduction, we will highlight the importance of psyllium seeds in the diet, provide basic information about psyllium seeds and their benefits, and give tips on how to use psyllium seeds in the kitchen.

Importance of psyllium in a healthy diet:

Psyllium seeds play an important role in promoting overall health and well-being. They contain soluble fiber that can help lower cholesterol, aid digestion, and keep blood sugar levels stable. By taking psyllium on a regular basis, many people can experience an improvement in their intestinal health, metabolism, and energy levels.

Basic information about psyllium and its benefits:

Psyllium seeds are the seeds of the psyllium plant, botanically known as Plantago ovata. Often referred to as "micronutrients" due to their small size, they are rich in fiber, omega-3 fatty acids and antioxidants. Their ability to bind water and swell gives them a gel-like consistency when in contact with liquid. This property makes them an excellent ingredient for thickening dishes or making gelatin substitutes in recipes.

The benefits of using psyllium seeds in cooking are many. They help regulate bowel movements, promote healthy intestinal flora, support weight management and reduce the risk of heart disease. In addition, they can help control blood sugar levels, lower cholesterol and reduce inflammation in the body.

Tips for using psyllium in the kitchen:

When it comes to using psyllium in cooking, there are some important tips to keep in mind. Here are some recommendations on how to incorporate psyllium into your meals:

Fluid intake: Psyllium seeds require sufficient fluid to develop their gel-like consistency. Be sure to drink enough water or other liquids when consuming psyllium to avoid expansion in the digestive tract.

Soaking: You can soak psyllium seeds before consumption to improve their swelling ability and increase their digestibility. Soak the seeds in water, yogurt or other liquids for about 10-15 minutes before using them.

Recipe ideas: Psyllium seeds can be used in recipes in a variety of ways. You can add them to smoothies, mueslis, yogurts, baked goods and even savory dishes like soups and sauces. Experiment with different recipes and discover new flavor combinations.

Dosage: Be sure to follow the recommended dosage of psyllium. Start with small amounts and gradually increase the amount to ensure that your body responds well.

Storage: Store psyllium seeds in a cool and dry place to maintain their freshness and quality. Close the package well to keep moisture and air out.

Conclusion:

Psyllium seeds are a valuable ingredient in cooking that offers numerous health benefits. Due to their fiber, omega-3 fatty acids and antioxidants, they can support digestion, heart health and metabolism. With the tips above, you can easily incorporate psyllium seeds into your daily diet and reap their health benefits. Be creative and experiment with new recipes to discover the versatility of psyllium seeds in the kitchen.

Chapter 1: Breakfast ideas

Breakfast is an important meal to start the day full of energy. With psyllium you can give your breakfast a healthy and nutritious touch. Here are three delicious breakfast ideas with psyllium that are easy to prepare:

Psyllium muesli with fresh fruit

Ingredients:

1 cup oatmeal

2 tablespoons psyllium

1 cup almond milk (or other vegetable milk)

1 teaspoon honey or maple syrup (optional)

A handful of fresh fruit (e.g. berries, sliced banana, chopped apples)

Preparation:

- In a bowl, mix the rolled oats, psyllium seeds and almond milk. Stir well to ensure that the psyllium seeds are evenly distributed.

- Let the muesli sit for 10-15 minutes so that the psyllium seeds can swell.
- Add honey or maple syrup to taste to give the muesli a natural sweetness.
- Add the fresh fruit to the cereal and enjoy.

Psyllium Pancakes:

Ingredients:

1 cup flour (wholemeal or gluten-free)

1 tablespoon psyllium

1 teaspoon baking powder

1 cup vegetable milk

1 tablespoon coconut oil (melted)

1 teaspoon vanilla extract

Fresh fruit or maple syrup to serve

Preparation:

- In a large bowl, mix the flour, psyllium seeds and baking powder.

- Add the vegetable milk, melted coconut oil and vanilla extract. Mix everything well until you get a smooth dough.
- Heat a pan and melt some coconut oil in it.
- Pour batter into pan to form pancakes of desired size. Bake until golden brown on both sides.
- Serve the finished pancakes with fresh fruit or maple syrup.

Psyllium Chia Pudding:

Ingredients:

2 tablespoons psyllium

3 tablespoons chia seeds

1 cup almond milk (or other vegetable milk)

1 teaspoon honey or maple syrup (optional)

Fresh fruit and nuts for garnish

Preparation:

- In a bowl, mix the psyllium seeds, chia seeds and almond milk. Stir well to avoid lumps.

- Let the pudding sit for 10-15 minutes to allow the psyllium and chia seeds to swell.
- Add honey or maple syrup to sweeten the pudding, if desired.
- Pour the pudding into glasses or bowls and refrigerate for at least 2 hours or overnight.
- Garnish with fresh fruit and nuts before serving.

Enjoy these delicious psyllium breakfast ideas and start your day in a healthy and nutritious way!

Chapter 2: Appetizers and snacks

A healthy diet also includes delicious appetizers and snacks. Here are three simple and delicious recipes with psyllium that are perfect as appetizers or snacks:

Psyllium crispbread with avocado dip:

Ingredients for the crispbread:

1 cup ground psyllium

1 cup flaxseed

1/2 cup sunflower seeds

1/2 cup pumpkin seeds

1/2 teaspoon sea salt

1 teaspoon dried herbs (e.g. oregano, basil)

Ingredients for the avocado dip:

1 ripe avocado

Juice of half a lemon

1 clove garlic (pressed)

Salt and pepper to taste

Preparation:

- In a bowl, mix all the ingredients for the crispbread
- Spread the mixture evenly on a baking sheet lined with parchment paper and press down.
- Bake at 180°C in a preheated oven for about 20-25 minutes until the crispbread is golden brown and crunchy.
- While the crisp bread is cooling, cut the avocado in half, remove the pit and scoop out the flesh.
- Place the avocado flesh in a bowl and mix with lemon juice, garlic, salt and pepper. Mash with a fork or blender until smooth consistency.
- Break the crispbread into pieces and serve with the avocado dip.

Psyllium Energy Balls:

Ingredients:

1 cup dates
1/2 cup ground psyllium
1/2 cup oatmeal
1/4 cup almond butter
2 tablespoons honey or maple syrup
1 teaspoon vanilla extract
A pinch of salt

Optional: shredded coconut, chopped nuts or chocolate chips for rolling

Preparation:

- Soak the dates in warm water until they are soft. Then drain the water.
- In a blender, combine the dates, ground psyllium seeds, rolled oats, almond butter, honey or maple syrup, vanilla extract and salt.

- Work the mixture to a sticky consistency. If the mixture is too dry, add a little water.
- Form small balls and roll in coconut flakes, chopped nuts or chocolate chips as desired.
- Place the energy balls in the refrigerator for at least one hour to set.

Psyllium crackers with hummus:

Ingredients for the crackers:

1 cup ground psyllium

1/2 cup chia seeds

1/2 cup sesame seeds

1/2 teaspoon sea salt

1 teaspoon dried herbs (e.g. thyme, rosemary)

Ingredients for the hummus:

1 can chickpeas (drained)

2 tablespoons tahini (sesame paste)

Juice of half a lemon

2 cloves of garlic (pressed)

2 tablespoons olive oil

Salt and pepper to taste

Preparation:

- In a bowl, mix all the ingredients for the crackers.
- Spread the mixture evenly on a baking sheet lined with parchment paper and press down.
- Bake at 180°C in a preheated oven for about 15-20 minutes until the crackers are crispy.
- Meanwhile, puree all ingredients for the hummus in a blender or food processor until smooth.
- Serve the psyllium crackers with the hummus.
- Enjoy these delicious and healthy appetizers and snacks with psyllium and bring variety into your kitchen!

Chapter 3: Soups and salads

In this chapter, I present you with three delicious recipes for soups and salads that contain psyllium. These dishes are not only healthy, but also easy to prepare and offer a wealth of flavor and nutrients.

Psyllium Minestrone Soup:

Ingredients:

1 tablespoon olive oil

1 onion (diced)

2 cloves garlic (chopped)

2 carrots (diced)

2 stalks of celery (diced)

1 can chopped tomatoes

4 cups vegetable broth

1/2 cup ground psyllium

1 teaspoon dried Italian herbs

Salt and pepper to taste

1 cup cooked pasta (optional)

Preparation:

- In a large pot, heat the olive oil and sauté the onion until translucent.
- Add garlic, carrots and celery and sauté for another 5 minutes.
- Add chopped tomatoes, vegetable broth, ground psyllium seeds and dried herbs. Stir well and bring to a boil.
- Reduce the heat and simmer the soup for 20-25 minutes until the vegetables are tender.
- Season to taste with salt and pepper. Optionally add cooked pasta and simmer for another 5 minutes.
- Serve the psyllium minestrone soup hot and enjoy.

Psyllium salad with roasted vegetables:

Ingredients:

1 cup mixed vegetables (e.g. bell bell pepper, zucchini, eggplant), cut into cubes

2 tablespoons olive oil

1 cup ground psyllium

2 cups hot water

Juice of one lemon

Fresh herbs (e.g. parsley, basil), chopped

Salt and pepper to taste

Preparation:

- Preheat the oven to 200°C.
- Drizzle the vegetables with olive oil and spread on a baking sheet.
- Roast the vegetables in the oven for about 20-25 minutes, until soft and lightly browned.
- In a bowl, pour hot water over the ground psyllium seeds and allow to swell for 5-10 minutes.
- Pour off the excess water and add the swollen psyllium seeds to the roasted vegetables.
- Add lemon juice, fresh herbs, salt and pepper. Mix well.
- Let the psyllium salad cool and serve.

Psyllium Taboulé:

Ingredients:

1 cup bulgur
2 cups hot water
1/2 cup ground psyllium
Juice from 2 lemons
3 tablespoons olive oil
1 cucumber (seeded and diced)
2 tomatoes (diced)
1 bunch fresh parsley (chopped)
Salt and pepper to taste

Preparation:

- Put the bulgur in a large bowl and pour hot water over it. Cover and leave to swell for 10-15 minutes.
- Sprinkle the ground psyllium seeds over the swollen bulgur and mix well.
- Add lemon juice, olive oil, cucumber, tomatoes and parsley. Stir well until all ingredients are well combined.

- Season with salt and pepper and let the psyllium taboulé steep in the refrigerator for at least 30 minutes.
- Stir the taboulé again before serving and enjoy.
- Try these healthy and delicious psyllium recipes for soups and salads and bring a variety of flavors and nutrients to your meals!

Chapter 4: Main dishes - Vegetarian and Vegan

In this chapter, I present you with three delicious vegetarian and vegan main dishes that contain psyllium. These dishes are rich in nutrients, full of flavor, and offer a healthy alternative to meat-based meals. Let's get right to it!

Psyllium burger with colorful vegetables:

Ingredients:

1 cup cooked chickpeas

1/2 cup ground psyllium

1 onion, finely chopped

2 cloves garlic, chopped

1/4 cup fresh parsley, chopped

1 teaspoon ground cumin seeds

1 teaspoon paprika powder

Salt and pepper to taste

2 tablespoons olive oil

Burger buns and desired burger toppings (e.g. lettuce, tomatoes, onions, avocado).

Preparation:

- In a bowl, mash the cooked chickpeas with a fork.
- Add ground psyllium, onion, garlic, parsley, cumin, paprika, salt and bell pepper. Mix well until a solid mass is formed.
- Let the mixture rest in the refrigerator for about 30 minutes.
- Shape the mixture into burger patties.
- In a skillet, heat the olive oil and fry the burger patties on both sides until golden brown and crispy.
- Place the psyllium burgers on burger buns and garnish with your favorite toppings. Serve them hot and enjoy the delicious taste!

Psyllium Ratatouille:

Ingredients:

2 zucchini, sliced

1 eggplant, cut into cubes
1 red bell bell pepper, cut into strips
1 yellow bell bell pepper, cut into strips
1 onion, thinly sliced
2 cloves garlic, chopped
2 tablespoons olive oil
1 can chopped tomatoes
2 tablespoons tomato paste
1 teaspoon dried Italian herbs
Salt and pepper to taste
1/4 cup ground psyllium

Preparation:

- In a large pot, heat the olive oil and sauté the onion until translucent.
- Add garlic, zucchini, eggplant and bell bell pepper. Sauté, stirring occasionally, for 5-7 minutes until vegetables are lightly browned.
- Add chopped tomatoes, tomato paste, Italian herbs, salt, pepper and ground psyllium seeds. Stir well.
- Cover the pot and simmer the ratatouille over medium heat for about 20-25 minutes,

until the vegetables are soft and the flavors have combined.
- Serve the psyllium ratatouille as a main dish or side dish. It goes well with rice or fresh bread.

Psyllium curry with coconut milk:

Ingredients:

1 onion, chopped

2 cloves garlic, chopped

1 piece ginger, finely chopped

2 tablespoons curry powder

1 teaspoon cumin

1 teaspoon turmeric

1 can coconut milk

1 cup vegetable broth

2 carrots, sliced

1 sweet potato, diced

1 cup cauliflower florets

1/2 cup green peas

1/4 cup ground psyllium

Salt and pepper to taste

Fresh cilantro for garnish

Preparation:

- In a large pot, sauté the onion, garlic and ginger until golden brown.
- Add curry powder, cumin and turmeric. Stir well until the spices are fragrant.
- Add coconut milk and vegetable broth to pot and bring to a boil.
- Add carrots, sweet potato and cauliflower. Simmer over medium heat for about 15-20 minutes until vegetables are tender.
- Add green peas and ground psyllium seeds. Cook for another 5 minutes until the curry is slightly thickened.
- Season to taste with salt and pepper. Garnish the psyllium curry with fresh coriander and serve together with rice or naan bread.
- Try these delicious vegetarian and vegan main dishes with psyllium and enjoy healthy and nutritious meals!

Chapter 5: Main dishes - meat and fish

In this chapter, I present you with three delicious main dishes with meat and fish that contain psyllium. These dishes are both delicious and healthy, offering a variety of flavors and textures. Whether you are a meat or fish lover, you will find inspiring recipes that are easy to prepare.

Psyllium-crusted chicken fillet:

Ingredients:

2 chicken breast fillets

1/2 cup ground psyllium

1/4 cup grated parmesan

1 teaspoon paprika powder

1/2 teaspoon garlic powder

Salt and pepper to taste

2 tablespoons olive oil

Preparation:

- Preheat the oven to 200 degrees Celsius and lightly grease a baking dish.
- In a shallow bowl, mix together ground psyllium seeds, grated Parmesan cheese, paprika, garlic powder, salt and pepper.
- Brush the chicken breasts with olive oil and then turn them in the psyllium mixture to get an even crust.
- Place the breaded chicken breasts in the prepared baking dish and bake in the preheated oven for about 25-30 minutes, until golden brown and cooked through.
- Before serving, let the chicken rest for a few minutes, then slice and serve with side dishes of your choice.

Psyllium salmon with lemon herb crust:

Ingredients:

2 salmon fillets
1/4 cup ground psyllium

2 tablespoons finely chopped fresh herbs (e.g. parsley, dill, chives)

Juice and zest of one lemon

Salt and pepper to taste

1 tablespoon olive oil

Preparation:

- Preheat the oven to 180 degrees Celsius and lightly grease a baking dish.
- In a bowl, mix ground psyllium seeds, chopped herbs, lemon juice and zest. Season to taste with salt and pepper.
- Brush the salmon fillets with olive oil and then coat both sides with the psyllium and herb mixture.
- Place the breaded salmon fillets in the prepared baking dish and bake in the preheated oven for about 15-20 minutes, until the salmon is tender pink inside and crispy outside.
- Serve the psyllium salmon with side dishes such as rice, potatoes or vegetables. Enjoy the fresh taste of lemon and herbs.

Psyllium meatballs with lean beef:

Ingredients:

500 g lean beef, minced
1/2 cup ground psyllium
1 onion, finely chopped
2 cloves of garlic, finely chopped
1 egg
2 tablespoons chopped parsley
1 teaspoon paprika powder
Salt and pepper to taste
2 tablespoons olive oil

Preparation:

- In a bowl, mix ground beef, ground psyllium, chopped onion, garlic, egg, chopped parsley, paprika, salt and bell pepper.
- Knead the mixture well until all ingredients are well combined.

- Form small patties and place on a baking sheet lined with parchment paper.
- Let the psyllium meatballs rest in the refrigerator for about 30 minutes to firm them up a bit.
- Heat a pan with olive oil and fry the meatballs in it until golden brown on both sides and cooked through.
- Serve the psyllium meatballs as a main dish with a side dish of your choice, such as mashed potatoes or salad.

Try these versatile main dishes with meat and fish containing psyllium and enrich your meals with the health-promoting properties of psyllium. Bon appetite!

Chapter 6: Side dishes and side salads

In this chapter I present you three delicious side dishes and side salads with psyllium. These dishes are perfect to complement your main dishes and provide extra nutrients and fiber. They are easy to prepare and add a healthy and delicious touch to your meals. Try these psyllium recipes for side dishes and let them convince you of their taste and health benefits.

Psyllium Mashed Potatoes:

Ingredients:

4 large potatoes, peeled and diced

2 tablespoons butter or vegetable margarine

1/4 cup milk or vegetable milk

1 tablespoon psyllium

Salt and pepper to taste

Preparation:

- Bring the diced potatoes to a boil in a pot of water and cook until tender, about 15-20 minutes.
- Drain the cooked potatoes and return them to the pot. Add the butter or vegetable margarine and mash with a potato masher or fork until you get a creamy consistency.
- Slowly add the milk or vegetable milk and continue mashing until the mashed potatoes are smooth.
- Stir in the psyllium seeds and season with salt and pepper. Serve the mashed potatoes warm and enjoy as a delicious side dish to your favorite dishes.

Psyllium Vegetable Rice:

Ingredients:

1 cup basmati rice

1 3/4 cups vegetable broth

1 tablespoon psyllium

1 tablespoon olive oil

1 onion, finely chopped

2 cloves garlic, chopped

Mixed vegetables of choice (e.g. carrots, peas, peppers), diced

Salt and pepper to taste

Preparation:

- Rinse the basmati rice thoroughly under running water to remove excess starch.
- Bring the vegetable broth to a boil in a saucepan and add the rice. Reduce the heat and simmer the rice, covered, until it is cooked and has absorbed the liquid.
- While the rice is cooking, heat the olive oil in a pan and fry the chopped onion until translucent. Add the garlic and fry for another 1-2 minutes.
- Add the diced vegetables to the pan and sauté, stirring occasionally, until tender.
- Add the cooked rice and psyllium to the vegetables in the pan. Mix everything well and season with salt and pepper.

- Serve the psyllium vegetable rice warm and enjoy as a healthy side dish to meat, fish or vegetarian main courses.

Psyllium Cucumber Salad:

Ingredients:

1 large cucumber, peeled and cut into thin slices
1 tablespoon psyllium
2 tablespoons Greek yogurt or vegetable yogurt
1 tablespoon lemon juice
1 teaspoon honey or maple syrup
Fresh herbs to taste (e.g. parsley, dill), chopped
Salt and pepper to taste

Preparation:

- Place the cucumber slices in a bowl and sprinkle the psyllium seeds on top. Mix well so that the psyllium seeds are evenly distributed.

- In a separate bowl, mix the Greek yogurt, lemon juice and honey or maple syrup. Add fresh herbs and season with salt and pepper.
- Pour the yogurt mixture over the cucumbers and psyllium and stir gently so that all ingredients are well combined.
- Let the psyllium cucumber salad steep in the refrigerator for about 30 minutes to allow the flavors to develop.
- Serve the refreshing psyllium cucumber salad as a side dish with a variety of dishes or enjoy as a healthy snack.
- These psyllium side dishes and side salads are not only delicious, but also healthy and high in fiber. They perfectly complement your meals and provide extra nutrients and flavor. Try these easy recipes and discover the versatility of psyllium in the kitchen.

Chapter 7: Snacks

In this chapter I present you three delicious and healthy snacks with psyllium. These snacks are perfect to keep your energy level up and satisfy your hunger between meals. They are easy to prepare and can easily be taken on the go. Try these delicious psyllium recipes and enjoy them any time of the day.

Psyllium Protein Bar:

Ingredients:

1 cup dates, pitted

1/2 cup almonds

1/4 cup psyllium

2 tablespoons cocoa powder

2 tablespoons protein powder (optional)

2 tablespoons maple syrup or honey

1 teaspoon vanilla extract

Pinch of salt

Preparation:

- Blend all ingredients in a high-powered blender or food processor until well combined and turned into a sticky paste.
- Pour the mixture onto a baking pan lined with parchment paper or a shallow bowl and spread evenly.
- Press the dough firmly together and place in the refrigerator to chill for at least an hour.
- Cut the chilled dough into bars and store in an airtight container in the refrigerator. Enjoy these nutritious psyllium protein bars as a quick snack or before or after a workout.

Psyllium Smoothie:

Ingredients:

1 banana, peeled and cut into pieces

1 cup frozen berries (e.g. strawberries, blueberries, raspberries)

1 cup spinach or kale

1 tablespoon psyllium

1 cup vegetable milk (e.g. almond milk, oat milk)

Optional: 1 tablespoon almond butter or peanut butter for added flavor and creaminess.

Preparation:

- Place all ingredients in a blender and blend on high speed until a smooth consistency is achieved.
- Pour the psyllium smoothie into a glass and enjoy immediately. You can garnish it with fresh fruit or nuts as you like.

Psyllium yogurt with fruits:

Ingredients:

1 cup Greek yogurt or vegetable yogurt (e.g. soy yogurt)

1 tablespoon ground psyllium seeds

1 tablespoon honey or maple syrup

Fresh fruit of your choice (e.g. berries, sliced banana, chopped mango)

Preparation:

- Pour the yogurt into a bowl and add the ground psyllium seeds. Stir well to distribute them evenly.
- Drizzle the honey or maple syrup over the yogurt and stir again to add a sweet note.
- Add the fresh fruit to the psyllium yogurt and gently fold in.
- Serve the psyllium yogurt with fruit immediately and enjoy as a refreshing snack.
- These delicious psyllium snacks are a healthy alternative to unhealthy snacks and provide you with important nutrients. Try them and let them convince you of their versatility and variety of flavors.

Chapter 8: Recipes for toddlers

In this chapter you will find three simple and healthy recipes with psyllium, especially suitable for young children. These dishes are nutritious and delicious, and psyllium seeds add extra fiber and healthy ingredients to your little one's diet. Try these kid-friendly psyllium recipes and treat your little ones to healthy treats.

Psyllium Oatmeal:

Ingredients:

1/4 cup oatmeal

1 cup water

1 tablespoon psyllium

A pinch of cinnamon (optional)

Fruits or berries for garnish (optional)

Preparation:

- In a saucepan, bring the water to a boil.

- Add the oat flakes and psyllium seeds and stir well.
- Reduce the heat to low and simmer the oatmeal, stirring occasionally, until it reaches the desired consistency (about 5-7 minutes).
- Add a pinch of cinnamon to taste and stir.
- Put the psyllium oatmeal in a bowl and garnish with fresh fruit or berries if desired.

Psyllium pasta with vegetable sauce:

Ingredients:

1 cup whole wheat pasta (e.g. whole wheat pasta or spaghetti)

1 tablespoon psyllium

Vegetables of choice (e.g. carrots, peas, peppers), washed and cut into small pieces

1 cup strained tomatoes

1 teaspoon olive oil

A pinch of dried herbs (e.g. basil, oregano)

A pinch of salt

Preparation:

- Cook the whole wheat pasta according to the instructions on the package until al dente. Drain and set aside.
- In a pan, heat the olive oil and sauté the cut vegetables until soft.
- Add the strained tomatoes, psyllium, dried herbs and a pinch of salt. Stir well and bring to a boil.
- Reduce heat and simmer vegetable sauce until slightly thickened (about 10-15 minutes).
- Add the cooked pasta to the vegetable sauce and mix gently so that the sauce is evenly distributed.
- Serve the psyllium pasta with vegetable sauce on a plate.

Psyllium Banana Pancakes:

Ingredients:

1 ripe banana, mashed

1 egg

2 tablespoons oat flour

1 tablespoon psyllium

A pinch of cinnamon (optional)

Coconut oil or butter for frying

Preparation:

- In a bowl, combine the mashed banana, egg, oat flour, psyllium and a pinch of cinnamon. Stir well until all ingredients are well combined.
- Heat a pan and melt some coconut oil or butter in it.
- Pour the batter into the pan in batches and form small pancakes.
- Fry the pancakes on both sides until golden brown and firm.
- Stack the psyllium banana pancakes on a plate and garnish with fresh fruit or a little honey, if desired.
- These recipes are quick to prepare and provide your toddlers with a healthy meal rich in fiber. Enjoy these delicious psyllium dishes with your little ones and encourage their healthy eating from the start.

Chapter 9: Sweet treats and desserts

In this chapter you will find three delicious and healthy recipes for sweet treats and desserts with psyllium. These dishes are ideal for satisfying your sweet tooth without sacrificing healthy nutrition. Psyllium seeds are a wonderful addition to desserts as they are rich in fiber and provide a natural source of healthy nutrients. Try these easy and tasty psyllium recipes and enjoy sweet temptations in a healthy way.

Psyllium Blueberry Muffins:

Ingredients:

1 cup whole wheat flour

1/2 cup psyllium

1 teaspoon baking powder

1/2 teaspoon salt

1/2 teaspoon cinnamon

1/4 cup honey or maple syrup

1/4 cup unsweetened applesauce
1/4 cup vegetable milk (e.g. almond milk)
1 teaspoon vanilla extract
1 cup fresh blueberries

Preparation:

- Preheat the oven to 180 degrees Celsius and line a muffin tin with paper cups.
- In a large bowl, mix together the whole wheat flour, psyllium seeds, baking powder, salt and cinnamon.
- In a separate bowl, whisk together the honey or maple syrup, applesauce, plant-based milk and vanilla extract.
- Add the wet ingredients to the dry ingredients and mix gently until a uniform dough is formed. Do not stir too long.
- Gently fold the fresh blueberries into the batter.
- Divide the batter evenly among the muffin cups and bake in the preheated oven for about 20-25 minutes, until the muffins are golden brown and firm.

- Remove the psyllium blueberry muffins from the oven and let cool completely before serving.

Psyllium apple pie:

Ingredients:

2 apples, peeled, cored and cut into thin slices
1 teaspoon lemon juice
1 cup whole wheat flour
1/2 cup psyllium
1 teaspoon baking powder
1/2 teaspoon cinnamon
1/4 teaspoon salt
1/4 cup honey or maple syrup
1/4 cup unsweetened applesauce
1/4 cup vegetable milk (e.g. oat milk)
1 teaspoon vanilla extract

Preparation:

- Preheat the oven to 180 degrees Celsius and grease a round baking dish.
- Place apple slices in a bowl and drizzle with lemon juice to keep them from browning.
- In a large bowl, combine the whole wheat flour, psyllium seeds, baking powder, cinnamon and salt.
- In a separate bowl, whisk together the honey or maple syrup, applesauce, plant-based milk and vanilla extract.
- Add the wet ingredients to the dry ingredients and mix well until a uniform dough is formed.
- Pour half of the batter into the prepared baking dish and smooth it out.
- Place the apple slices evenly on the dough.
- Pour the remaining batter over the apple slices and smooth.
- Bake the psyllium apple pie in the preheated oven for about 25-30 minutes, until golden brown and firm.
- Remove the cake from the oven and let it cool before cutting it into pieces and serving.

Psyllium chocolate pudding:

Ingredients:

2 ripe avocados
1/4 cup unsweetened cocoa
1/4 cup maple syrup or date syrup
1 teaspoon vanilla extract
1 tablespoon psyllium
Pinch of salt
Fruits or nuts for garnish (optional)

Preparation:

- Cut the avocados in half, remove the pit and scoop the flesh out of the skin with a spoon.
- Place the avocado in a blender or food processor and puree until smooth.
- Add the unsweetened cocoa, maple syrup or date syrup, vanilla extract, psyllium and a pinch of salt.
- Mix everything well until a creamy consistency is reached.

- Pour the psyllium chocolate pudding into bowls or glasses and chill in the refrigerator for at least 1 hour to set.
- Garnish with fresh fruit or nuts as desired before serving.
- Enjoy these sweet treats and desserts with psyllium in moderation and enrich your meals with healthy and fiber-rich options. Your family will love these delicious creations while benefiting from the health benefits of psyllium.

Chapter 10: Drinks with psyllium

In this chapter you will find refreshing and healthy drink recipes with psyllium. These drinks are not only delicious, but also a great way to incorporate psyllium into your daily diet. Try these easy psyllium drinks and enjoy them any time of the day.

Psyllium Smoothies:

Ingredients:

1 ripe banana

1 cup frozen berries (e.g. strawberries, blueberries, raspberries)

1 tablespoon psyllium

1 cup vegetable milk (e.g. almond milk, oat milk)

Optional: sweetener as needed (e.g. honey, maple syrup)

Preparation:

- Peel the banana and cut into pieces.

- Place all ingredients in a blender and blend to a smooth consistency.
- Add sweetener if needed and blend again.
- Pour the psyllium smoothie into a glass and serve immediately.

Psyllium Iced Tea:

Ingredients:

2 bags of herbal tea (e.g. peppermint tea, chamomile tea)

1 tablespoon psyllium

4 cups water

Lemon slices (optional)

Ice cubes (optional)

Optional: sweetener as needed (e.g. honey, agave syrup)

Preparation:

- Bring the water to a boil and add the tea bags. Let the tea brew for about 5 minutes.
- Remove the tea bags and allow the tea to cool.

- Pour the cooled tea into a pitcher or carafe.
- Add the psyllium seeds and stir well.
- Add lemon slices and ice cubes to taste.
- If necessary, add sweetener to taste and stir.
- Pour the psyllium iced tea into glasses and serve chilled.

Psyllium lemon water:

Ingredients:

1 tablespoon psyllium

1 lemon

4 cups water

Ice cubes (optional)

Optional: sweetener as needed (e.g. honey, stevia)

Preparation:

- Squeeze the juice from the lemon and set aside.
- Pour the water into a pitcher or carafe.

- Add the psyllium seeds and lemon juice to the water and stir well.
- If necessary, season with sweetener and stir again.
- Add ice cubes to chill the drink.
- Pour the psyllium lemon water into glasses and serve immediately.

Enjoy these refreshing psyllium drinks as a healthy alternative to sugary beverages. They are easy to prepare and provide an extra portion of fiber in your diet. Try different variations and find your personal favorite psyllium drink.

Chapter 11: Psyllium for external use

In this chapter you will discover the versatile use of psyllium seeds for external application. In addition to incorporating psyllium into your meals, you can also use these small seeds for natural skin and hair care treatments. Here are three simple recipes for psyllium face mask, psyllium hair care mask and psyllium body scrub.

Psyllium face mask:

Ingredients:

1 tablespoon ground psyllium seeds

1 teaspoon honey

2 teaspoons natural yogurt

Preparation:

- Place the ground psyllium seeds in a bowl.
- Add the honey and the natural yogurt.

- Mix all ingredients thoroughly until a uniform paste is formed.
- Thoroughly clean and dry the face.
- Apply the psyllium face mask to the face, avoiding the eye area.
- Leave the mask on for about 15-20 minutes.
- Then rinse the mask with warm water and gently dry the face.

Psyllium hair care mask:

Ingredients:

2 tablespoons ground psyllium seeds

1 ripe avocado

1 tablespoon olive oil

Preparation:

- Cut the avocado in half, remove the pit and place the flesh in a bowl.
- Add the ground psyllium seeds and olive oil.
- Thoroughly mix all ingredients together until a creamy consistency is achieved.

- Wash the hair thoroughly and dry lightly.
- Apply the psyllium hair care mask to the entire hair, paying special attention to the ends.
- Cover the hair with a shower cap or towel and leave the mask on for about 30 minutes.
- Then rinse the hair thoroughly with warm water and style as usual.

Psyllium body scrub:

Ingredients:

3 tablespoons ground psyllium seeds

2 tablespoons coconut oil

1 teaspoon honey

Optional: essential oil of choice (e.g. lavender oil, lemon oil)

Preparation:

- Warm the coconut oil slightly until it is liquid.

- Put the ground psyllium seeds in a bowl and add the liquid coconut oil.
- Add the honey and, if necessary, the essential oil.
- Mix all ingredients thoroughly until a homogeneous mixture is obtained.
- Apply the body scrub to damp skin in the shower or bath.
- Massage the body with gentle circular movements to remove dead skin cells and stimulate blood circulation.
- Rinse the scrub thoroughly and gently dry the skin.

These psyllium applications for external use offer a natural and gentle way to care for your skin and hair. Enjoy the many benefits of psyllium seeds and pamper your body externally with these homemade beauty treatments.

Chapter 12: Recipes for pets

Your beloved pets can also benefit from the health benefits of psyllium. In this chapter, I present you with three easy recipes for psyllium treats for dogs, psyllium cat cookies, and a psyllium food supplement for rodents. These homemade treats are not only tasty, but also nutritious for your furry friends.

Psyllium treats for dogs:

Ingredients:

1 cup oatmeal

1/2 cup peanut butter (unsweetened and without xylitol)

2 tablespoons ground psyllium seeds

1/4 cup water

Preparation:

- Preheat the oven to 180 degrees Celsius and line a baking tray with baking paper.

- Place the rolled oats, peanut butter and ground psyllium seeds in a bowl.
- Add the water and mix all ingredients thoroughly until a dough is formed.
- Shape the dough into small balls and place on the prepared baking sheet.
- Bake the treats in the preheated oven for about 15-20 minutes until golden brown.
- Allow the treats to cool completely and then give them to your dog as a reward or snack.

Psyllium Cat Cookies:

Ingredients:

1/2 cup tuna (in water)

1 egg

1 tablespoon ground psyllium seeds

1/2 cup whole wheat flour

Preparation:

- Preheat the oven to 180 degrees Celsius and line a baking tray with baking paper.

- Drain the tuna and place in a bowl.
- Add the egg and mix everything well.
- Add the ground psyllium seeds and whole wheat flour and mix thoroughly again until a dough is formed.
- Roll out the dough on a lightly floured surface and cut out small cookies in any shape.
- Place the cookies on the prepared baking sheet and bake in the preheated oven for about 10-12 minutes, until firm and crisp.
- Let the cookies cool completely and then offer them to your cat as a treat.

Psyllium food supplement for rodents:

Ingredients:

1 tablespoon ground psyllium seeds

1 teaspoon dried herbs (e.g. parsley, chamomile)

1/4 cup rodent food (e.g. pellets or seed mixture)

Preparation:

- Place the ground psyllium seeds in a small bowl.
- Add the dried herbs and mix well.
- Add the rodent food and mix thoroughly again so that the psyllium and herbs are well distributed.
- Store the food additive in an airtight container and add to the rodent food as needed. Make sure that your pet has enough fresh water available.

These simple recipes allow you to provide your pets with the valuable nutrients of psyllium in a healthy way. Treat your furry companions to these delicious and nutritious treats and food supplements. However, always consider the individual needs and preferences of your pets and consult your veterinarian if necessary.